CONTENTS

INTRODUCTION

Pneumonia is the single largest infectious cause of death in children globally, killing more than 2,500 children a day worldwide. It's also to blame for up to 7 percent of all deaths in adults. According to the American Lung Association, believe it or not there are more than 30 different causes of pneumonia. Luckily not every case is very serious or life-threatening, especially those considered to be "walking pneumonia," a milder type that rarely requires serious intervention or hospitalization to deal with pneumonia symptoms.

The most common cause of pneumonia infections is complications due to other respiratory illnesses, especially the flu. Other reasons you or your child might come down with pneumonia? These include contact with certain fungi or viruses, catching pneumonia from someone's who infected, or even exposure to indoor air pollution and toxic chemicals.

The severity of pneumonia symptoms that someone experiences depends on factors like the specific type of pneumonia the person has (bacterial versus viral), medical history, age and strength of the immune system. If you have viral pneumonia, unfortunately you also are at risk for getting bacterial pneumonia too — making pneumonia symptoms even worse and complications more likely.

What can you do to help lower your odds of developing pneumonia, especially if you already have several other risk factors like a history of lung damage, smoking or other respiratory problems? The first step is to eliminate any voluntary risk factors that increase your chances of catching bacterial infections or viruses in the first place — especially suffering from nutrient deficiencies, leaving illnesses untreated and cigarette smoking.

WHAT IS PNEUMONIA?

Pneumonia is a type of respiratory infection that affects the lungs. Pneumonia infections can be bacterial or viral, which partially determines the type of pneumonia symptoms that someone develops due to having the illness.

Initially when someone develops pneumonia, symptoms are about the same whether the infection is caused by bacteria or a virus (these normally include mild fever, a dry cough, headache, muscle pains and fatigue/weakness). Feverish symptoms tend to get worse however within several days when the pneumonia infection is bacterial in nature. Most people start to display more severe pneumonia symptoms within about three days of the infection taking hold, including having trouble breathing, coughing up mucus and developing higher fevers. In some cases, viral pneumonia causes more symptoms than bacterial cases do, although each person is different.

Is pneumonia contagious? Yes, pneumonia can spread from person to person, but it can also develop in other ways too.

The same types of bacteria or viral pathogens that cause pneumonia infections are already present in many people's airways and sinuses (especially in children, who carry these organisms in their noses and throats). The real problem starts when these organisms enter and infect the lungs. How strong someone's immune system is largely determines whether or not these organisms have the chance to spread, proliferate and cause an acute lung infection, which is exactly why improving overall immunity is the best way to protect yourself or your children.

TYPES OF PNEUMONIA

The severity of the infection depends on many factors, including your age and overall health.

"A lot of treatment aspects, as well as outcome, depend on the person, as well as the type of pneumonia they have," says Dr. Barron. "Sometimes you'll be fine just resting, but if you have things like trouble breathing, you should get to a doctor right away."

Knowing the cause of a lung infection is important for determining which type of pneumonia you have, how you got it, and how to treat it.

Here's what you need to know about the different types of pneumonia:

Community-Acquired Pneumonia

Also known as CAP, this is the most common form of pneumonia because you can catch it in public places, such as at school or work. It can be caused by bacteria, viruses, or fungi.

You can also develop CAP after you get a common viral infection, such as a cold or the flu.

The illness ranges from mild to serious and, if left untreated, can lead to respiratory failure or death.

Bacterial CAP is usually more serious than other types and is more common among adults. Atypical pneumonia, often called walking pneumonia, is a milder form.

Viral and bacterial pneumonia share some common signs, but doctors can often distinguish between them by a patient's symptoms.

Various types of bacteria are responsible for the illness. In most cases, the bacteria will enter the lung during inhalation, but it can also go through the bloodstream if other parts of the body are infected.

Streptococcus pneumoniae, also known as pneumococcal pneumonia, can be treated with antibiotics. But according to the CDC, many type's of bacteria, including some S. pneumoniae (pneumococcus), are resistant to those antibiotics, which can lead to treatment failures. Pneumococcal pneumonia causes up to 175,000 hospital admissions a year in the United States.

You can also have a pneumococcal infection without having pneumonia. For example, pneumococcal infections also cause more than three million ear infections in children every year.

Risk factors for bacterial CAP include:

- Having an underlying lung disease, like asthma or COPD
- Having a systemic disease, such as diabetes
- Having a weakened immune system
- Being very young or very old
- Being disabled
- Abusing alcohol
- Smoking

Depending on how sick you are and whether or not you have any other health conditions, your doctor may treat you for bacterial pneumonia with antibiotics either at home or in the hospital.

Viral CAP, particularly the respiratory syncytial virus (RSV), is the most common cause of pneumonia in children younger than two years old.

Although viral pneumonia is generally less severe than bacterial pneumonia, viral infections caused by certain flu viruses, such as severe acute respiratory syndrome (SARS), can be very serious.

Antibiotics are ineffective against viral pneumonia. Your doctor will most likely treat the symptoms — fever, cough, and dehydration.

You or your child may need to be hospitalized if your viral pneumonia symptoms become severe.

Fungal CAP is most common in people with an underlying health problem or a weakened immune system, including those with HIV or AIDS and people undergoing treatment for cancer. It's treated with antibiotics or antifungal medication.

Getting a vaccination against pneumococcal pneumonia reduces your risk for CAP.

Healthcare-Associated Pneumonia

This refers to an infection that develops in someone being cared for in a healthcare facility, such as a hospital or nursing home. If you've been hospitalized or admitted into a long-term nursing or rehab facility, you may be at risk for more deadly forms of pneumonia.

Symptoms of this type of pneumonia are more serious and may include shortness of breath, high fever, and chest pain.

Hospital-Acquired Pneumonia

As the name suggests, this develops during a hospital stay for a different health problem. People who are on machines to help them breathe are particularly prone to developing hospital-acquired pneumonia.

Hospital-acquired pneumonia usually needs to be treated in the hospital with intravenous antibiotics.

Aspiration Pneumonia

This can develop after a person inhales food, liquid, gases, or dust.

A strong gag reflex or cough will usually prevent aspiration pneumonia, but you may be at risk if you have a hard time swallowing or have a decreased level of alertness.

A form of aspiration pneumonia, chemical- or toxin-related pneumonia is caused by the inhalation of chemical fumes, as through an exposure to a mix of ammonia and bleach, or in the breathing in of kerosene or some other noxious chemical.

This type of pneumonia can also occur in older people with poor swallowing mechanisms, such as stroke victims, who actually can inhale the acidic contents of their stomachs, causing aspiration pneumonia.

This causes inflammation without bacterial infection. These pneumonias can sometimes be difficult to treat, especially because the patients are sicker to begin with.

Once your lungs have been irritated by breathing in food or stomach contents, a bacterial infection can develop.

Some conditions that may put you at risk for aspiration pneumonia include:

- Overuse of drugs or alcohol
- Seizure
- Head injury or anesthesia
- Gastroesophageal reflux disease (GERD)
- Various neurological diseases
- Chronic lung disease, such as COPD

Symptoms of aspiration pneumonia include cough, increased sputum, fever, confusion, and shortness of breath.

Treatment may include breathing assistance and intravenous antibiotics given in the hospital.

You can prevent complications by not eating or drinking before surgery, working with a therapist to learn how to swallow without aspirating, and avoiding heavy use of alcohol.

IS PNEUMONIA CONTAGIOUS?

Most types of bacterial pneumonia are not highly contagious. Even though it is possible to spread bacteria from one person to another, pneumonia typically occurs in people with risk factors or weakened immune defenses when bacteria that are normally present in the nose or throat invade the lung tissue. Any kind of bacterial or viral pneumonia has the potential to be contagious, but Mycoplasma pneumoniae and Mycobacterium tuberculosis (the cause of tuberculosis) are two types of bacterial pneumonia that are highly contagious. Breathing in infected droplets that come from patients who are coughing or sneezing can spread the disease to others.

HOW LONG IS PNEUMONIA CONTAGIOUS?

It is impossible to say with certainty exactly how long an adult or child with pneumonia is contagious, since this varies according to the type of germ or organism that caused the pneumonia. This contagious period can range from one to two days to weeks. In general, while an infected person is coughing or sneezing, there is the potential to release contaminated droplets into the air.

Many bacterial pneumonias are much less contagious after antibiotics have been taken for about 24-48 hours. However, this time period may vary for some organisms. For example, with tuberculosis, it can take two weeks or more of antibiotics before the person is no longer contagious. With viral pneumonias, the patient becomes less contagious after the symptoms have improved, especially fever. Some people with viral pneumonia may not be contagious after one to two days with no fever, but others may still shed some infectious virus particles for a much longer time.

PNEUMONIA SYMPTOMS AND SIGNS

The most common signs and symptoms of pneumonia are:

Persistent coughing, sometimes which can become painful

Coughing up mucus — sometimes mucus can contain small amounts of blood or appear green and/or yellow

Trouble breathing normally and shortness of breath — wheezing is more common when the pneumonia is viral

Chest pains, especially when moving around and breathing more heavily

Developing a fever — usually fevers are mild but in some people become high (in cases of bacterial pneumonia, fevers can sometimes cause body temperature to rise to almost 105 degrees F), and in the case of bacterial pneumonia, it can take several days for fevers to become severe

Experiencing other symptoms of a fever, such as having the chills, headaches, stomach aches, confusion/disorientation, shaking or sweating

Fatigue and sometimes muscle aches

Nausea, upset stomach or loss of appetite

Sometimes rapid heartbeat, rapid breathing, changes in skin color and becoming delirious, especially when experiencing a high fever

In infected infants, serious complications can sometimes develop, including being unable to drink, unconsciousness, hypothermia and convulsions

Wondering about symptoms of walking pneumonia exactly and if it's also contagious? Walking pneumonia is a non-medical term to describe a mild case of pneumonia, usually caused from bacteria in the lungs. Most cases of walking pneumonia are due to a bacterial microorganism called Mycoplasma pneumonia, which is contagious and spread just like other types of pneumonia.

PNEUMONIA CAUSES AND RISK FACTORS

How do you get pneumonia exactly, and who has the highest risk of developing this illness?

Pneumonia is caused by a variety of infectious agents and develops when the lungs become filled with pus and mucus, making it hard to breathe, get enough oxygen and control coughing. The parts of the lungs that are most affected by pneumonia infections are called the alveoli, which are small sacs that normally fill up with air/oxygen and allow for someone to breathe properly.

While people of all ages and levels of health can develop pneumonia for many different reasons, researchers believe that there are five main infectious agents to blame that are the primary causes of pneumonia:

Certain types of harmful bacteria, which lead to infection of the lungs. These most commonly include Streptococcus pneumonia (especially in children with pneumonia) and Haemophilus influenzae type b. Pneumocystis jiroveci is another type of bacteria that's associated with death due to pneumonia in children with viruses, such as HIV.

Certain types of viruses. This type of pneumonia is often called respiratory syncytial virus.

Mycoplasma, which contributes to walking pneumonia most often.

Infection due to other organisms, including fungi.

Exposure to certain toxic chemicals (such as from fumes, tobacco products or cigarettes) that weaken the immune system.

Infectious agents that cause pneumonia can be transmitted from person to person or spread from certain parts of someone's body (like the nose) to the lungs. Some of the ways these agents are passed include someone:

Inhaling them. Organisms can be spread via airborne droplets.

Being near someone else who is infected and coughing or sneezing.

Being exposed to blood from someone with pneumonia.

Pregnancy and delivery. If the mother is infected, the infant can become infected after being exposed to her blood.

RISK FACTORS FOR PNEUMONIA INCLUDE

Becoming infected with the flu or another respiratory infection/virus (such as a cold, laryngitis, bronchitis or influenza)

Having any chronic respiratory or lung disease, such as COPD or cystic fibrosis

Being an older adult — research shows that the elderly tend to suffer from pneumonia and experience more serious complications than younger adults

In children, having any form of chronic respiratory disease or frequent respiratory infections, especially COPD, severe allergies or asthma

In infants, if their mothers were infected or have another respiratory illness they can become infected too

Having a weakened immune system due to other illness like autoimmune disorders, viruses such as HIV, measles, hepatitis or serious infections

Malnutrition, lack of safe drinking water or undernourishment due to a poor diet

Taking certain medications that lower immunity

In infants, being formula-fed instead of breast-fed, which improves immunity

Smoking cigarettes and having related complications, such as lung damage or emphysema

Having difficulty swallowing (due to a history of other medical problems, such as suffering from a stroke, dementia, cerebral palsy or Parkinson's disease)

A history of common inflammatory diseases that weaken the immune system, including diabetes, heart disease or liver disease/damage

Living or spending lots of time in tight quarters, especially if unhygienic, where you're in close contact with other infected people (this can include nursing homes, day cares, etc.)

Exposure to air pollution, both inside and outside — indoor air pollution can be caused from parents smoking or burning/heating with biomass fuels

Recovering from surgery or trauma

WHAT TESTS DIAGNOSE PNEUMONIA?

The diagnosis of pneumonia always begins with taking a medical history and performing a physical examination to look for characteristic signs. In particular, listening to the lungs may reveal areas where sound is diminished, wheezing, or crackling sounds in affected areas. Some commonly performed diagnostic tests are as follows:

A chest X-ray is able to illustrate whether or not pneumonia is present, but it does not provide information about the organism responsible for the infection.

In some cases, a chest CT scan may be performed. This will reveal more detail than the chest X-ray.

Pulse oximetry measures the amount of oxygen in the bloodstream. The test involves a painless sensor attached to the finger or ear. Blood levels of oxygen may be reduced in pneumonia.

Microbiology tests to identify the causative organism. Tests may be performed on blood or sputum. Rapid urine tests are available to identify Streptococcus pneumoniae and Legionella pneumophila. Cultures of blood or sputum not only identify the responsible organism but can also be examined to determine which antibiotics are effective against a particular bacterial strain.

Bronchoscopy is a procedure in which a thin, lighted tube is inserted into the trachea and major airways. This allows the doctor to visualize the inside of the airways and take tissue samples if needed. Bronchoscopy may be performed in patients with severe pneumonia or if pneumonia worsens despite antibiotic treatment.

CONVENTIONAL TREATMENT FOR PNEUMONIA SYMPTOMS

Treatment for pneumonia depends on its cause, specifically if it's bacterial pneumonia or viral pneumonia. According to the World Health Organization (WHO), "Pneumonia can be prevented by immunization, adequate nutrition, and by addressing environmental factors. Pneumonia caused by bacteria can be treated with antibiotics, but only one third of children with pneumonia receive the antibiotics they need."

The type of oral antibiotic that's most commonly used to treat bacterial pneumonia is called amoxicillin, which is usually given in tablet form. Remember that viruses cannot be cured with antibiotics, so in this case the patient must overcome the illness by waiting and managing symptoms. Most people don't require hospitalization unless complications develop, such as a very high fever, or it's an infant who's infected. In recent years, vaccines have also been introduced for certain types of pneumonia, specifically those that target and the pneumococcal conjugate type.

As you'll learn, there are also many natural ways you can protect yourself from the different pathogens that cause pneumonia. Today, most of the focus regarding pneumonia is on prevention since this is the best way to keep complications and transmission from causing widespread problems. Not relying on antibiotics also lessens the risk globally for antibiotic-resistant pneumonia.

PREVENTION AND NATURAL TREATMENTS FOR PNEUMONIA SYMPTOMS

1. Improve Immune Function

Limiting your exposure to other people with the infection, while at the same time boosting immune strength, is the best way to control pneumonia transmission and is critical for both prevention and treatment. Steps you can take to immediately reduce your risk for infections or viruses include:

Improving your diet and gut health — Avoid inflammatory or common allergenic foods like processed grains, gluten, conventional dairy products, lots of added sugar, processed foods with synthetic ingredients and sweetened beverages with artificial flavors.

Taking probiotic supplements — Probiotics help populate the GI tract with healthy bacteria that actually keep bad bacteria in check. You can also get probiotics from your diet naturally by eating probiotic foods like cultured veggies and yogurt.

Getting enough sleep — Aim for seven to nine hours per night.

Exercising — the benefits of exercise include improving immune function, helping prevent infections and lowering inflammation.

Managing stress — Stress can increase inflammation, weaken the immune system and make infectious symptoms last longer than necessary.

Other immune-boosting supplements — these include vitamin C, astragalus root, licorice root, echinacea, garlic, turmeric and ginger, which can speed up healing. There are also other antiviral herbs that keep you protected from future infections and recurrences.

2. Breast-feed Infants

One of the best ways to prevent pneumonia infections in infants and children is to exclusively breast-feed them during the first year of life, followed by providing adequate nutrition during their earliest years. This has been shown to help protect young children from numerous illnesses beyond pneumonia too, including allergies and asthma.

In addition to breast-feeding babies, risk for infection and mortality due to pneumonia during infancy or childhood is greatly reduced when children aren't malnourished and have access to safe drinking water and sanitary living/school environments. Avoiding exposure to secondhand smoke, preventing indoor air pollution, treating food allergies, preventing nutrient deficiencies and keeping up with doctors' appointments can all keep your baby or child safe.

3. Manage Fever Symptoms

To help keep a fever from getting worse or a high fever from causing further complications, here are tips that you can implement at home:

Suck on ice cubes or make homemade ice pops to prevent dehydration.

Take cooling baths or showers, or wrap a damp, chilled towel around your neck. You can also soak a towel in peppermint oil for extra cooling effects, thanks to its natural menthol.

Drink chilled/iced peppermint, thyme or chamomile herbal tea.

Get enough electrolytes by making homemade green or fruit smoothies' or from drinking coconut water.

Get plenty of rest and sleep.

Take an over-the-counter fever reducer if symptoms become very bad, such as ibuprofen or Advil.

4. Control Coughing Naturally

Consume mucus-reducing foods to naturally treat coughs or wheezing, including homemade vegetable soups, bone broth and green tea.

Breathe in moist, warm air as much as possible, avoiding very cold temperatures.

Rub on a topical cough suppressant or use natural cough syrup made with essential oils like eucalyptus, thyme, cedar wood, nutmeg, camphor and peppermint.

Avoid strenuous workouts that can make shortness of breath or chest pain worse.

Clean your home regularly to remove irritants, inhale or diffuse essential oils, and try using a humidifier.

5. Practice Good Hygiene and Reduce Household Air Pollution

Clean up dust mites, pet hair and other common allergens (especially if someone in the family suffers from asthma symptoms).

Prevent pneumonia from spreading by washing your hands regularly with soap (ideally the kinds made with natural ingredients that fight bacteria).

Don't smoke indoors or burn toxic fumes when cooking or heating your home.

Inhaling gases and contact with construction debris should also be avoided at work.

Reduce your use of household products made with strong chemicals, instead using natural cleaning products to help clean surfaces, fabrics and even your skin.

Very drastic temperature changes, humidity, high temperatures or extreme cold might all make pneumonia symptoms worse, so try to avoid these situations.

PNEUMONIA STATISTICS AND FACTS

The WHO reports that pneumonia results in more than 920,000 deaths in children each year. This accounts for roughly 15 percent of all deaths of children under the age of 5 years old.

It's also to blame for up to 7 percent of all deaths in adults, or more than 4 million deaths annually.

People in every nation develop pneumonia, but the infection is most prevalent in underdeveloped nations, especially parts of South Asia and sub-Saharan Africa.

People living in underdeveloped nations develop pneumonia up to five more often than those living in industrialized nations do. India, China, Pakistan, Bangladesh, Indonesia and Nigeria are currently the nations with the highest prevalence rates of pneumonia.

Worldwide over $109 million is spent annually in antibiotics to treat pneumonia infections.

Infants and children under 4 years old or elderly adults who are over 75 are most at risk for developing pneumonia.

Of around 450 million total cases of pneumonia per year, about 200 million are due to viral strains of the infection.

In the U.S. alone every year, approximately 1.86 million emergency visits are due to pneumonia.

Between 20 percent to 40 percent of people with pneumonia visit the hospital and require hospitalization.

More than $10 billion is spent in the U.S. annually to treat pneumonia infections and complications, making it one of the most expensive conditions to manage for the health care system.

Pneumonia occurs during the winter months more than any other time of the year, similar to the flu.

Males tend to get pneumonia more often than females do, and African-Americans tend to suffer more commonly than Caucasians.

PNEUMONIA VS. WALKING PNEUMONIA

Because walking pneumonia is usually milder than other cases, symptoms are normally less severe and sometimes not even very noticeable at all.

While pneumonia commonly causes symptoms like fatigue, fever, the need for bed rest or sometimes even hospitalization, some people with walking pneumonia are able to carry on with their regular routines for the most part, although they're still contagious.

It's believed that during "outbreaks" of walking pneumonia, which occur every several years on average, this type accounts for about half of all pneumonia cases.

Walking pneumonia is usually caused from bacterial infection due to mycoplasma. It affects people living or working in tight quarters most often, since it's usually transmitted through tiny airborne droplets, passed from sneezing or coughing.

People with walking pneumonia are generally contagious for about 10 days, even when they don't show symptoms.

Higher prevalence rates for walking pneumonia have been reported among school-aged children, military recruits and adults younger than 40 who live in places like homeless shelters, prisons, or crowded and unsanitary buildings. People living in nursing homes or staying in the hospital are also at risk for all types of pneumonia.

Compared to more severe cases of pneumonia that are most common during the winter, walking pneumonia usually peaks in prevalence during the late summer months.

NUTRITION IN PNEUMONIA

Patients with pneumonia have a great risk of having an altered nutritional status, I recommends the following nutritional tips to help in the recovery process while ensuring that nutritional deterioration does not occur. As the first step of management of pneumonia, the patient should be guarded against vomiting, if present.

Food intake: What to eat, what to avoid

Patient's with pneumonia have increased energy needs due to the elevated body temperature and accelerated metabolism associated with the difficulty in breathing. Such patient's should be encouraged to increase their intake with nutrient-rich foods, vitamins, and minerals.

Patients with pneumonia should maintain the intake of adequate calories to keep the nutritional status from deteriorating and subsequent prevention of malnutrition.

The body of the patient requires more nutrients once the treatment for pneumonia has been initiated to repair the damaged tissue. There is a significant risk of increased recovery time if the patient is malnourished. An adequate diet that is rich in calories, protein and micronutrients are highly recommended.

Foods that are dense in vitamin A should be recommended for patients with pneumonia as it helps maintain the integrity of the respiratory mucosa. Patients should focus on beta carotene foods that are generally yellow or orange in their natural color like carrot, apricots and papaya. Also, green leafy vegetables like spinach and kale are great.

Foods containing starches and saccharine should be avoided.

Fluid intake

The loss of fluid in pneumonia caused by diarrhea and/or sweating is associated with an increased need for fluid. Therefore, these patients should have sufficient provision of liquids. This can be in the form of soups, juices or infused water.

As long as fever persists in patients, fluids should be extensively given to the patient. Solids, if given, should be very nourishing and easily digestible. Fresh juices of fruits and vegetables are highly recommended for patients with pneumonia.

PNEUMONIA IN CHILDREN

Pneumonia is an infection in one or both lungs. Pneumonia can be caused by bacteria, viruses, fungi, or parasites. Viruses are usually the cause of pneumonia in children. Children with viral pneumonia can also develop bacterial pneumonia. Often, pneumonia begins after an infection of the upper respiratory tract (nose and throat). This causes fluid to collect in the lungs, making it hard to breathe. Pneumonia can also occur if foreign material, such as food or stomach acid, is inhaled into the lungs.

DISCHARGE INSTRUCTIONS:

Return to the emergency department if:

- Your child is younger than 3 months and has a fever.
- Your child is struggling to breathe or is wheezing.
- Your child's lips or nails are bluish or gray.
- Your child's skin between the ribs and around the neck pulls in with each breath.
- Your child has any of the following signs of dehydration:
- Crying without tears
- Dizziness
- Dry mouth or cracked lip
- More irritable or fussy than normal
- Sleepier than usual
- Urinating less than usual or not at all
- Sunken soft spot on the top of the head if your child is younger

than 1 year

- Contact your child's healthcare provider if:
- Your child has a fever of 102°F (38.9°C), or above 100.4°F (38°C) if your child is younger than 6 months.
- Your child cannot stop coughing.
- Your child is vomiting.
- You have questions or concerns about your child's condition or care.

Medicines:

Antibiotics may be given if your child has bacterial pneumonia.

NSAIDs, such as ibuprofen, help decrease swelling, pain, and fever. This medicine is available with or without a doctor's order. NSAIDs can cause stomach bleeding or kidney problems in certain people. If your child takes blood thinner medicine, always ask if NSAIDs are safe for him or her. Always read the medicine label and follow directions. Do not give these medicines to children under 6 months of age without direction from your child's healthcare provider.

Acetaminophen decreases pain and fever. It is available without a doctor's order. Ask how much to give your child and how often to give it. Follow directions. Read the labels of all other medicines your child uses to see if they also contain acetaminophen, or ask your child's doctor or pharmacist. Acetaminophen can cause liver damage if not taken correctly.

Ask your child's healthcare provider before you give your child medicine for his or her cough. Cough medicines may stop your child from coughing up mucus. Also, children under 4 years old should not take over-the-counter cough and cold medicines.

Do not give aspirin to children under 18 years of age. Your child could develop Reye syndrome if he takes aspirin. Reye syndrome can cause life-threatening brain and liver damage. Check your child's medicine labels for aspirin, salicylates, or oil of wintergreen.

Give your child's medicine as directed. Contact your child's healthcare provider if you think the medicine is not working as expected. Tell him or her if your child is allergic to any medicine. Keep a current list of the medicines, vitamins, and herbs your child takes. Include the amounts, and when, how, and why they are taken. Bring the list or the medicines in their containers to follow-up visits. Carry your child's medicine list with you in case of an emergency.

FOLLOW UP WITH YOUR CHILD'S HEALTHCARE PROVIDER

Write down your questions so you remember to ask them during your visits.

Help your child breathe easier:

Teach your child to take a deep breath and then cough. Have your child do this when he or she feels the need to cough up mucus. This will help get rid of the mucus in the throat and lungs, making it easier to breathe.

Clear your child's nose of mucus. If your child has trouble breathing through his or her nose, use a bulb syringe to remove mucus. Use a bulb syringe before you feed your child and put him or her to bed. Removing mucus may help your child breathe, eat, and sleep better.

Squeeze the bulb and put the tip into one of your baby's nostrils. Close the other nostril with your fingers. Slowly release the bulb to suck up the mucus.

You may need to use saline nose drops to loosen the mucus in your child's nose. Put 3 drops into 1 nostril. Wait for 1 minute so the mucus can loosen up. Then use the bulb syringe to remove the mucus and saline.

Empty the mucus in the bulb syringe into a tissue. You can use the bulb syringe again if the mucus did not come out. Do this again in the other nostril. The bulb syringe should be boiled in water for 10 minutes when you are done, and then left to dry. This will kill most of the bacteria in the bulb syringe for the next use.

Keep your child's head elevated. Ask your child's healthcare provider about the best way to elevate your child's head. Your child may be able to breathe better when lying with the head of the crib or bed up. Do not put pillows in the bed of a child younger than 1 year old. Make sure your child's head does not flop forward. If this happens, your child will not be able to breathe properly.

Use a cool mist humidifier to increase air moisture in your home. This may make it easier for your child to breathe and help decrease his or her cough.

How to feed your child when he or she is sick:

Bottle feed or breastfeed your child smaller amounts more often. Your child may become tired easily when feeding.

Give your child liquids as directed. Liquids help your child to loosen mucus and keeps him or her from becoming dehydrated. Ask how much liquid your child should drink each day and which liquids are best for him or her. Your child's healthcare provider may recommend water, apple juice, gelatin, broth, and popsicles.

Give your child foods that are easy to digest. When your child starts to eat solid foods again, feed him or her small meals often. Yogurt, applesauce, and pudding are good choices.

WHAT ARE THE SIGNS AND SYMPTOMS OF PNEUMONIA IN THE ELDERLY?

As with many diseases and illnesses, the signs and symptoms vary from one person to the next and may mimic other disorders too. In general terms, the following are common signs and symptoms of pneumonia in the elderly.

Confusion – In elderly people, pneumonia can cause confusion or disorientation. They may complain about having a hard time thinking or seem addled when trying to explain or do things that are normally not challenging for them. This type of symptom mimics other diseases such as dementia and can be a result of medications so it is hard to diagnose pneumonia based on this symptom. However, any change in mental status should be reported to a doctor or in a facility, to a medical professional, such as the charge nurse.

A Productive Cough – Typically, moist and wet sounding coughs that produce phlegm. You may also hear audible wheezing as the person inhales and exhales. These symptoms also mimic the common cold and the flu. The general rule of thumb is that a cold with a fever should be evaluated, especially for the elderly.

Fever – There are various types of pneumonia and some may only produce a low-grade fever in the 99°F – 100°F range while others may produce fevers above 101°F. Fevers often include sweating and shaking, both of which is the body's natural response to being overheated. A fever that lasts more than 24 hours should be evaluated.

Chest Pain and Rib Pain – Pneumonia can be painful on a couple of levels.

First, there is often rib pain because of the chronic coughing. In the elderly, heavy coughing can fracture ribs and potentially cause spinal problems, such as slipped disk and vertebra alignment issues. In addition, the added fluid in the lungs means that people either have to pant or take deep breaths and breathing deeply can be painful. Rapid breathing or panting is a serious symptom and should be evaluated immediately. Generally, it means that the surface area of the lungs are covered and the remaining lung tissue must do more work to supply vital organs with oxygen. This often coincides with pale and clammy skin. Panting is a sign of many life-threatening illnesses such as heart attack, congestive heart failure, and shock. These symptoms should always be evaluated immediately.

Fatigue – Pneumonia is a draining illness that saps elderly people leaving them exhausted. That tiredness comes from many aspects of the illness. First, it takes a lot of energy for a body to fight off an illness. It can also increase the risk of falls and secondary injuries.

Fever, which is heat, burns a lot of energy just like a furnace. The higher the heat setting the more fuel it burns. There is a lot of physical labor with pneumonia too. Coughing, rapid breathing, and the struggle to do anything all take up a vast amount of energy. That energy drain can rob the immune system of the energy it needs to do its job. The lack of oxygen also contributes to fatigue. As the body shuttles oxygen to the most important organs it leaves the muscles starved and weak. This weakened state puts elderly people at risk for compound injuries, such as falling, broken hips, and sprains.

As mentioned, the symptoms of pneumonia vary from one person to the next and change based on the health level of the person who is inflicted. Those with chronic disease have the hardest time, but pneumonia can be deadly even in the healthiest of our elders.

HOW MANY PNEUMONIA VACCINES DO YOU NEED?

PCV13 or Prevnar 13, is currently recommended for all children younger than 2 years of age, all adults 65 years of age or older, and people 2-64 years of age with certain medical conditions.

PPSV23 is currently recommended for all adults 65 years of age or older and for people who are 2 years of age or older and at high risk for pneumococcal disease (for example, those with sickle cell disease, HIV infection, or other immunocompromising conditions). PPSV23 is also recommended for use in adults 19-64 years of age who smoke cigarettes.

There is no evidence about the safety of PCV13 or PPSV23 vaccine use in pregnancy. Women who need the vaccine should be vaccinated before a pregnancy, if possible.

Some people may be recommended to receive both the PCV13 and PPSV23 vaccines. The U.S. Centers for Disease Control and Prevention (CDC) recommends two pneumococcal vaccines for all adults 65 years or older. The PCV13 and PPSV23 should not be given at the same time. When both vaccines are recommended, a dose of the PCV13 should be given first, followed by a dose of PPSV23 at another visit to a health care provider.

Seasonal influenza vaccines are available yearly and are recommended to decrease the chance of contracting influenza. Vaccines against the measles virus and varicella virus, two viruses that can also cause pneumonia, are also available. The common side effects of these vaccines are similar to those listed below for the pneumonia vaccine.